Quit Overcomplicating Fitness: Guide to Go from Geek to Gladiator

Jesse Chapman

TABLE OF CONTENTS

Prologue

My name is Jesse Chapman, I'm 18 years old, I grew up in a small town in the depths of southeastern Virginia. Oh wait, you thought the American Psycho style opening was what I was going with, you know, the one that includes the insane daily routines of perpetual exercise 7 days a week with thousands of stomach crunches and other kinds of laboring work? No, that's not the case by far. I used to believe this, I used to agree and train hard in the gym with weights for 7 days a week and would also utilize cardio training in my regime. However, no significant results were made to achieve the body of my dreams. I knew fitness took time and that muscles need a great extent of said time to grow and shape properly in an aesthetic format, yet no matter what I did it was like fighting an uphill battle with no end in sight. This left me straggled and isolated with a pit of disappointment in my stomach. I wanted to look like my idols, first it was Daniel Craig, the actor who plays James Bond, next it was Hugh Jackman, the iconic Wolverine star, and also internet fitness icons such as Jeff Seid, Zyzz, and Connor Murphy. These guys had a presence whenever they walked into a room. Women would want them and men would want to be them. For someone like me who had always been viewed by his peers as the "cringeworthy, awkward, unattractive kid," I was looking for an escape from that stereotype and into the world of my role models, dreaming of looking as chiseled as a Greek statue, seeking a higher level of confidence, and gaining respect from girls. Not only did I change my attitude towards my goals to achieve such things, I decided, under the guidance of my trainer, Kevin Parrott, to quit overcomplicating so many things regarding fitness. This includes, but isn't limited to training style, diet, preparation, rest, etc. This shift in mindset led to a shift in my physique, as I have successfully transformed my body from weak and skinny fat to that of a ripped gladiator. If one reads and follows this guide to less stress, less over complication, and more free time to spend reaping the benefits of your work in the gym, then there is no doubt that your life will change and that you will earn the respect that you have craved for ages. So without further ado, let's get started!

Chapter 1

Goal in Mind

When I started my fitness journey, I had a complete and well thought out goal in mind. I was going to make all the girls who had rejected and friend zoned me extremely jealous and wishing they could take back the way they had treated me. I wanted them to see me with a body like Daniel Craig in the iconic role of James Bond. Maybe then, I pondered, they would give me another chance and shot at a relationship with them. I beat it in my head that I was going to train everyday, a concept that is highly flawed, but kept me in the state of mind for the achievement of the goal I set forth so that I would never stop or waver no matter what got in my way. On a daily basis I would rewatch the iconic shirtless scene from Casino Royale and just envision myself walking around with a body as good as that. All in all, once I achieved a great physique, those girls did return and attempt to rekindle their previous times with me, but at that point I had moved on, I had visualized and was maximizing myself to my greatest potential, not letting anyone stop or slow me down.

I say this to bring up the question to you, the reader, what is your goal? Why do you want it so bad? How will you achieve it? What will you do when you achieve it? So many people grow impatient when their body goal doesn't happen in an instant amount of time. More often than not it takes months or even years to achieve your goal. People that tell you fast routes to get shredded or buff are just full of it and are trying to scam and take your money. That's all it is. No matter who it is, if they offer you a shortcut, avoid it at all costs, because it's not even worth your time. Consider this, if I showed up to you with a bag of donuts in my hand and said to pay me $500 for you to eat them and you'll instantly have a Ferrari or Aston Martin because of the special ingredients, would you believe me? Of course not! That is exactly what a lot of these fitness experts do with their supplements and such, they hide ineffective ingredients and sell you an overpriced product and laugh all the way to the bank. Never trust these people. They will never get you to your goal of a dream body, rather they will slow you down.

Another point that I want to bring up is your motivation. More than likely it's to pick up girls. I mean who doesn't want that. Your body plays a big factor, but its not everything. Once you fall in love with training and the bodybuilding lifestyle, you don't necessarily want a long term relationship with someone, but rather you want respect from women. I always used to hate when I would hang out with girls and they would totally salivate over a more strong and fit guy than I was at the time. That is just a major shot to your confidence. So once I started to train, not only did I have this motivation in mind to change it, but I was determined and zeroed in to make sure that wouldn't happen again. Now, I have a large circle consisting of many girls that admire and respect the way that I work and train. I have gained such a large amount of respect from them due to this mentality and zeal that I possessed to achieve the goal that I had set forth for myself. Apply that style of mentality to your fitness goal. Just everyday take time out and think about what it will be like to achieve what you have set forth to achieve. Once you make it there, it is so fulfilling, you'll never want to stop your diet and training. At that point, it doesn't become a chore or task, it becomes a lifestyle you've adapted to.

So the last, but most important thing I wish to ask is this, what is your goal? This is vital to determine as it is what will guide you through the ups and downs of the next years of your life. Keep in mind that some goals simply aren't naturally attainable. If you want to look like Ronnie Coleman or Jay Cutler in a month naturally, then sorry, that's not going to happen. Think realistically and plan accordingly. Set benchmarks for yourself to meet and surpass over time. You never want to leave any of your potential on the table. It's not complicated at all, if you want to look like a Hollywood actor, what's stopping you? Laziness and procrastination will never yield you anything. It will just push off your dreams until they become forgotten and you accept your fate as a person who failed to get to their aspirations. Nobody wants to be that person. Visualize your goal, then constantly think about it over and over, especially when those feelings of laziness and procrastination start to creep in. I did this with my fitness goals myself. I remember one time when I sat there and thought of not going to the gym one day, then all of a sudden, I decided to get off my butt and go there because I thought, "Hugh Jackman would never quit on the gym, why should I?" Thinking like that boosted me through the many strong and weak points. You'll never stagnate with that mindset, remember that.

Finishing this chapter, remember to never let any distraction deter you off the path to your dream physique. It's really not complicated. Willpower is overhyped because most people are too incompetent to even give it a try. View this as a challenge. Set what you have in mind for the future and go out and get it. The only person stopping you is yourself. The potential is endless. Go get it tiger!

Chapter 2

Getting Started

Congratulations, you have a pretty epic body goal in mind! You already just took the first step by thinking about your goal that you want to achieve. Way to go! Time for you to get started towards achieving your goal. Stay committed, have endurance, but above all, be as consistent in what I share with you as you possibly can. Let's go!

First things first, either you need a membership to a local gym or if you have the adequate equipment at home, you can workout there. Personally, I prefer to go out to the gym as it motivates you to get out the house and do something instead of slacking because if the gym is in your house, right next to the couch, you may decide to choose that latter because you can do the lifting "anytime." In reality, you have less excuses to workout at home than any other place, but I digress. I attend a 24 hour gym regularly, that way I can show up whenever and still get the necessary workout in rather than pushing it off because of the gym being closed. 24 hour gyms, while maybe having lesser equipment, are better to get you in the   mindset of getting in shape and achieving your goal as the place never stops or slows down. Franchises that I recommend, and keep in mind that I'm not even paid to sponsor them, are Snap Fitness, One Life, and Anytime Fitness. Once you sign up for the membership, immediately start going, don't procrastinate, you aren't just going to wake up with your goal being there.

If you're training in a gym style format, here's some of the best advice I can offer, never "ego-lift", don't approach women to hit on them while they're working out, and lastly avoid grunting or drawing extra attention to yourself when you're working out. Ego lifters, in my opinion, are the worst to deal with when you are trying to train for aesthetics. I see them all the time in my own gym, lifting heavy weights with improper movements and incredibly poor form. I honestly don't know what these people expect to get out of it. I mean it's not like they will ever change or improve themselves if they can't even do the exercise properly. Plus, all that heavy weight combined with bad form is really going to kill their joints in the future. Avoid training with people like this as much as possible, they won't ever bring you up, all they will do is pull you farther away from where you want to be. Never forget, it's not how much you lift, its how much you look like you lift. Train with weights that challenge you, but you can achieve proper form with. Then and only then will you reach the goals you have set forth for yourself.

Ever see that cringey guy at a party, you know, the one that goes out of his way to find the most attractive girl in the room, only to awkwardly approach her and make her and everyone around uncomfortable due to his lack of game and horribly awful timing. Well that is who you will be in the gym if you try to hit on somebody while they're training. I know, we all are trying to get with an attractive fitness girl, or even get them to notice us, but going out of your way to get their number or hit on them really isn't going to help your chances at all, in fact, it will blackball you from getting that opportunity ever again. You are going to lose confidence and likely avoid the gym and her like the plague because of that feeling of humiliation and embarrassment. Instead, stay in your own lane, this isn't the club or the bar, just workout, diet properly, and stay zeroed in on the prize. Likely, if she's a consistent attendee herself, she'll start to notice you more and you will gain a great rapport that may spring into something better, who knows, anything is possible. Remember, all good things take time, once she sees you all jacked in the gym she is the one that will be coming to you rather than you going to her. It's a very simple process. Train hard, eat clean, and reap the benefits of your hard work. It's totally worth it.

What's worse than being a total dork in front of girls in the gym is being a total dork in front of everyone. It's quite a task, but believe me, it happens more often than not. So many guys go in the gym acting like they're hot stuff, grunting during reps, dropping weights, or doing other things that literally everyone in the gym facepalms and gets uncomfortable around. You are supposed to act like a stud when you're training, not an escaped gorilla from the zoo. This sort of behavior is typical of the cocky gym rat, similar to that of an ego lifter, never adapt to the way that this kind of person trains. All it will do is drag you down with them. Believe me, gym cred is a hard thing to earn, but horrible to lose and try to get back. There's some things that people won't ever let anyone live down and that is a sad fact. One of those is being a dunce in the gym. For the love of all things holy, remember that, and don't get tripped up and become someone different than who you are.

In conclusion, getting started is a big step, but if you follow this gym etiquette code that I have written above for you, there is no way you can't succeed. You will gain so many friends and the admiration of others through this process. It's definitely a system that I can personally attest to that has worked for me over   the past couple of years. I made my fair share of mistakes through it, however, I learned and am trying to help you avoid the same kinds of faults and missteps that I made over that period of time. I want to leave you with this. Remember, getting started is a great beginning, however unless you adapt these habits and codes consistently, you won't maximize your full potential. Remember the bylaws and advice above and you will go far.

Chapter 3

Discipline and Consistency of a Gladiator

I hate the society clichés of how a diet or a workout regime is "so hard" to stay consistent with. I mean seriously, every T.V. show or movie promotes this lazy, juvenile idea, thus making viewers subconsciously apply this mentality in their own lives. This vast majority of society gets a sort of vindication from these sources that a lack of diligence and gumption to stick with something is somehow acceptable in today's world. But you, the reader, you aren't like regular people. If you read this far, you know that you are a warrior in the making. So proceeding onward, in order to earn those stripes, remember, one of the essential components in the foundation of a warrior is your consistency and discipline regarding your regime and goals.

It's hard to get out of a bad habit, no matter if the habit is gluttony, drinking, or smoking. However, the fastest breakthrough to your freedom is a simple discipline and change of routine. When you start attending the gym and dieting, begin to slowly roll back the unhealthy behaviors that you had previously been   partaking in. Cold turkey solutions are temporary, ease yourself into a routine by just having more healthy behaviors than unhealthy ones. Slowly cutting them out until there are none left will significantly help you adjust your lifestyle. The gradual change will better help you to adapt to the new foods and exercises that you are putting your body through. One by one and day by day you will witness so many changes to your physique to the point that you will be so proud of yourself and your stick to it mentality that you won't even crave or want to reminisce of your previous style of living. This is the style of a gladiator, envision yourself getting there, plan accordingly, and then there is nothing stopping you from reaching it.

The big concept to never forget though is to not lose consistency in your plans that you set for yourself. Sure it's okay to treat yourself occasionally, but when occasionally becomes frequently, that's when it becomes a mega problem. Fitness is a lifelong thing, by making such a commitment to your health and wellbeing, not only do you benefit your life, but those around you as well. When people start to see the first signs of progress, not only will they aspire to your level of physique, but their jaw will drop as they witness and view the consistency of your training. Even those that brush off your accomplishments, deep down, they still desire to know how you got there and what your secrets were. Embarking on this journey is a major maturity leap that some may never comprehend. You are a gladiator though, you understand it because you wish to live it. Your consistency is what makes you as a person. Imagine if you didn't consistently invest or go to school. You are likely to fail or be broke. The same mentality applies to fitness. It's a core concept to live by in all aspects of your life.

I personally have a love for the routine that I currently have. Without it my life wouldn't be as optimal as it is at the moment. There's no better feeling than waking up early, having near superhuman level focus, a great body similar to that of a Hollywood actor, or simply being noticed when you attend an event or walk into a room of people. My last routine before I started training was to sleep in late, play video games, eat fast food, come home, maybe hang out with friends, eat out again, and then sleep. It was rinse and repeat day in and day out. I hated that version of myself. I honestly got so sick of that way of living. I was just a regular person, never to be noticed by anyone. Nothing made me stand out. Following the methods above, I zeroed in on my goal and changed accordingly. It took time, but within a year and a half of consistency, I reached great milestones. Still, I'm not stopping there.

You control your life, don't let anything or anyone hold you back. Instant gratification is simply that, instant gratification. Sure, it may feel good to skip training or to eat something that is contrary to a fitness style of diet. However, while they are satisfying, they are short term moments that really don't bring the best out for the future, in fact, they may ruin your plans for your future dreams. Practice this mental exercise, think about the long term of every action you take, whether its menial or major. Think about how great you'll feel inside when you push off the short term moment of happiness for the long term goal of everlasting satisfaction. Continually do this on a weekly basis. After about 2 to 3 weeks, you will automatically have a great discipline. This exercise is a great starting point on the road to lifetime health and aesthetics. Practice this and other methods in this book and trust me, nothing will ever stop you or even get in your way on your road to success.

Chapter 4

Bulk or Cut?

Bulking and cutting is really the dumbest argument and strategy when it comes to building muscle. I hear the debates all the time, I see it in the forums, so I think that is fair to dispel this bodybuilding "bro-science." People bicker all the time about how bulking is "necessary" because the caloric surplus consistently over a long period of months is the key to gaining muscle mass and size. They say that it is the only way to gain a decent amount of mass the fastest and that it is a necessary component. Likewise, they regard cutting as vital as well. Dropping low in calorie intake to make the excess bulk fat go away to uncover the muscle. The fact of the matter is this, the body can only put on about 8-10 pounds of muscle a year! Bet you didn't see that coming, but it's true! Here is the concept that I adapt to gain muscle that doesn't require looking fat at some points of the year and lean other points, rather I maintain a ripped figure over the whole year in its entirety.

As a certified personal trainer, I know what has worked for me and it may possibly work for you as well. Anyhow, rather than bulking and putting on excess fat in my midsection and waistline, I follow this method instead. This method being to drop body fat first! I know, pretty contrary what most people do, but then again, most people don't have their dream bodies do they? By dropping levels of fat, especially once you reach the 10% threshold or lower, you will uncover the muscle that was beneath the previous layer of blubber that was covering it up. While you may not stand out in clothes initially, you'll be shredded and cut once you pop your shirt off. As you train consistently and diet well, you will begin to beef up over time. Trust me, 10 pounds more of muscle on a lean body is a way better look than 10 pounds on a fatter, bulkier body. Plus on a bulkier physique, if they wanted to lean down, the caloric deficit could suppress or eliminate the muscle they've gained and built over the past hard year, making their hard work and effort come out on the wash, as they may only be able to retain 3-6 pounds of muscle they've worked for.

Don't just take my word for this, look at former Mr. Olympia, the Father of Aesthetics, Frank Zane. Zane, known for his not overly massive, but proportional physique and build quoted in an interview once that one should, "never bulk up." It makes plenty of sense to me. Why would a former Mr. Olympia be deceptive over such a controversial training topic such as this? Most people in the fitness industry that discuss this subject are always trying to sell you something. Maybe it's a "fast growing muscle supplement" or a "bulk-up quick starter kit." Just remember, as stated in an earlier chapter, that these claims are all false and are exaggerated to a crazy extent. Never trust these advertisements and claims. Listen to trustworthy people and experiment on your own. Maybe different things work for different individuals and that is a possible case, however, just think rationally about these approaches, and choose the one that seems the most rational and effective as the facts are presented. Not only just the facts of effectiveness, but the facts of what is likely a healthier thing to do that will prolong and make your life more enjoyable.

Recapping this chapter, be contrary to what the major concepts are in the fitness industry. If the bulking and cutting cliché was the end all be all, why does it look like so many people never got out of the bulk phase? Seriously! I see so many guys day in and day out that have been training for years trying to get that beach body they want, yet they don't even look like they train. The excessive bulk fat is keeping these individuals from popping out in public with their shirt on, or at the beach with their shirt off. Not trying to pick on these guys, I'm just using them as an example to illustrate that the bulk mentality simply does not apply to everybody. It's just a fact, If you want to truly transform from weak to warrior, not only does it require the discipline and consistency discussed in the previous chapter, it also requires having the nerve to be unique and outside of the box. Why would you want to be like everyone else? No matter if its fitness or in personal matters, always cut your own path and be different from what you're expected to be. Society never wanted you to get ripped, they wanted you to look like everyone else. They wanted you to shut up about your dreams and get back to school and work to repeat the same overbearing and boring tasks day in and day out. They want you to be average. That may work for some people, but not people like us. Forget what the world wants from you. Forget what the fitness industry expects you to do. Be your own person. Adapt that mentality, that's how you know that you are leaving the weak mindset and becoming a gladiator!

Chapter 5

Training

There are so many dumb, baseless, and inaccurate misconceptions regarding the training style and format of many lifters and fitness types that have a great and aesthetic physique. The most common of these however is that these gifted and talented individuals must "slave for hours," or "workout every day of the week." These assumptions couldn't be farther from the truth. It doesn't take 2-3 hours in the gym on a day to day basis to make gains and progress towards where you dream to be. In fact, if you follow that method and style, not only will you likely quit and be burnt out with no social life whatsoever, but you will make very minimal progress if any at all. I know what you're thinking. "What? You mean it's not good to be in the gym all the time? I thought that was the lifestyle." No, training consistently is necessary, however, overtraining is the most detrimental thing you could ever do to your body.

Overtraining is a common rookie mistake, heck, I was the poster child for it. I lifted seven days a week to only slight avail. I had no set foundation or true plan of action. I would sort of just wing it every time I walked in and would just see where it all took me. At the time, it may have been for the good sole purpose of just getting my once lazy self into the gym, but as time went on, I was beginning to get heavily frustrated. I mean who wouldn't? You're constantly in the gym pushing your limits and have nothing to show for it! However, that didn't deter me. Applying the mentality and goal setting objectives that were mentioned in the previous chapters, I began to search for answers and to find ways to make the most of my efforts. More often than not, you find all of your answers when your back is against the wall. This story here is no exception. I searched and was blessed to find my trainer, Kevin Parrott, a longtime bodybuilder and major figure in the sport.

Upon my first consultation, I was given these three training keys that have significantly helped me and will likely help others achieve their fitness goals. These keys were to train only three days per week, train different body parts each day, and train to the point of hypertrophy and for muscle contraction. This totally locked in my training. I was earning the body of my dreams. It is a very bewildering concept to understand at first, believe me, I understand your confusion for sure. It's hard to believe that less frequency actually yields better results than more of it. I mean you know what they say in the old cliché, "less is more." I just had no clue that applied to more than just awkward social interactions.

The reason training three times a week is vital for the optimal gains of a true warrior is due to this simple concept. That being that resting and recovery is what builds muscle. I get so mad when people with the "bro-science" mentality always say their dumb sayings like "No Rest Days Bro!" These people fall into the classes of people that you should not trust or affiliate with in the gym. They can talk tough all they want, but their chicken legs and lack of training knowledge is what will keep you behind. Anyway, rest is key as that is where protein synthesizes and repairs the minor tears to muscle that you've made in your training, because that is simply what lifting does, it leaves minor tears in your muscle that are repaired. Thus, gaining a larger, more defined shape.

Along with training three days a week, it is important to remember to target different parts of the body each day that you train. This targeting of different muscles weekly will give your body enough time to rest. By training your body in this fashion, each muscle group will not only be better recovered, but it will be even fresher when you return the next week to hit the gym. This boost of energy is going to make each workout more productive and thoroughly more enjoyable. You will not only be fresher and focused in the gym, but you will also progressively be getting stronger. I personally recommend training chest, biceps, and forearms one day, legs and abs the next, and back, shoulders, and triceps the last day. It's normally best to leave one rest day in between each training day.

Training form is more important than the weight used. Use a weight that challenges you, but isn't overbearing to the point that there is possible injury. This emphasis on form is going to create hypertrophy and muscle contraction. These will create and initiate the muscle building process. This is where those little tears mentioned are created. By slowing down and contracting the muscle, you are properly executing the right form necessary to grow the muscle that you are training. Typically I use a slow negative motion on the third rep of my isolation exercises to ensure that the muscle I'm training is contracting, so as not to create a wasted motion.

All in all, combining all these elements and implementing the strategies above, you will no longer dread your training, rather you will look forward to it! Get started with this style of training!

Chapter 6

You Are What You Eat!

Great job so far! You're training hard and are getting pretty good gains so far, there's just another thing you have got to do in order to maximize this fitness journey. What is it you might ask? Changing your eating habits! You are what you eat! That's right, I just said it, so let's put down the Taco Bell quesadilla, we have much to discuss my friend.

The key to any noticeable change in one's body is a change in their diet. More often than not people misconstrue training to be the end all be all when it comes to ones lifelong fitness and health, and yes, training is very crucial, however, it's not the most important thing. It's commonly known that 60 to 80% of this process is controlled by the dietary habits of an individual. Diet is the biggest thing as the nutrients for the body and allow for muscle growth to occur and for one's fat loss to stimulate. Personally, I hate regarding things as diet, as diet is a dirty word for individuals just downing tasteless kale salads with nothing but crunchy, boring croutons at the top of it. What's worse is when people think of the word "diet" it rings a bell that they have to be at a point of near starvation to make any noticeable difference to their body. Both of these viewpoints are completely flawed and false.

To start off, don't refer to it as a "diet," rather refer to it as a meal plan. A meal plan programs your brain to view it as long term, while the word "diet" may only program you for the interim and brief period of time. Start by eating major carb sources such as rice, sweet potato, and whole wheat bread only in the early hours up to around 2 P.M. After that, your source of carbs should be in vegetable forms. Eating the major or what I refer to as "heavy" carb source too late in the day, may likely stunt your progress in losing body fat. Along with those carb sources, always have protein along with it. Examples of good protein sources that will build muscle are beef, chicken, steak, fish, and eggs. These are going to serve as the building blocks for muscle growth. Preferably, one should eat steak or beef as a lunch entree, as it may stick in their gut for too long a period if they consume it in the afternoon. In the afternoon though, that is where the fish and chicken come in. Always make sure they are both cooked grilled and with very little to no seasoning on it whatsoever. Seasoning make have excess sodium or added sugars which may make water weight stick to your core and make your face appear more bloated and less symmetrical. We don't want that to happen! You've worked way too hard for this!

Along with the high protein diet, be sure to consume water continuously throughout the day. Personally, a good starting point that I would recommend is for you to drink a gallon of water every day. It may seem like a lot at first, however, if you pace yourself and make it a point that by the time you get to sleep, that you have already consumed at least one gallon of water, then you will be set! Water is a magical thing really. What it does and why it is so important to muscle growth and fat loss is incredibly extraordinary! Water makes up 75% of the muscle and when more is consumed, the muscle building and recovery process is significantly bolstered, not only that, but the muscles appear fuller as well. Also, with a greater consumption of water taken in, you will be more vascular as well. I remember when I first started this, I saw veins that I didn't even knew I had! My body had flushed out the excess water weight covering it! When you steadily consume water, these are the miracles that happen! Incredible am I right? Start incorporating this as soon as possible, once one gallon is attainable, I recommend two gallons, but not an extra gallon after that. Even though water is a good thing, there's always problems with too much of a good thing. Too much water in excess may cause one to lose too many essential nutrients, but if you stay in these confines, you should be just fine.

In conclusion, your meal plan is your meal ticket to your goal physique. Even if you are unable to train one week, if you can keep your nutrition in check, you will be able to preserve your hard earned gains and understand what fuel you need to keep the body running and growing. Be persistent and diligent in your meal plan, if you don't start off doing well that is okay! It takes time to get used to things and to break free from previous rituals, routines, and habits. Take baby steps and before you know it, you will be dedicated to this meal plan. This not only teaches and trains you for the betterment of your physical health, but your mental health as well. You become trained to have maximum willpower and emotional strength. This strength that you learn from this journey will propel you through life and truly keep you ahead of all the others in the pack. Always strive for that such consistency! You'll achieve it for sure! I know so!

Chapter 7

Supplements

Okay, you're going to be bombarded with so much information about supplements as you begin this training process. I'm serious, brace yourself for those annoying YouTube and Facebook ads because they are going to be coming right at you. Just a fair warning. The key though is to really research the supplements that you are about to take before you use them. Promise me that you readers won't be the knuckleheads that believe everything that all those supplement companies claim their product does. More often than not if it sounds too good to be true, it probably is. I'm just being factual, if they claim to put mass and muscle on you within a week or so basis, than more than likely they are being boldface liars to you. Also, be very careful of the ingredients of the substance. Occasionally, there are news stories of illegal substances being slipped into the mix of the particular supplement. Not only is that sick and disgusting from a health perspective, but it punishes the consumers who may not know better. However, that won't be you, you're not just a strong, jacked gladiator, you're very wise as well. Listen close to all I mention, this chapter is very important.

Starting off, in the supplement industry, while there are many companies that have a proven track record of effectiveness that aid to create beneficial muscle gains, there are many that are just out there to make a buck. You may wonder how these lying and scam products from these companies are able to be sold online or in stores. The answer is simple, the supplement industry is one of the least regulated industries there is. Nearly no restrictions are placed on what is done to prepare or distribute these items. While this is extremely good in terms of vast and cheaper prices due to the competition in the marketplace, the dark side is that there is many of these companies, some being no name companies with a lack of a genuine reputation, place elements in their products that are either harmful or ineffective as the consumer and their use of the product is not the thing they care about at all. It is truly sickening what all these people get away with. Always research the products and companies that they are affiliated with before you buy them! Supplements are expensive, don't let these greedy cowards con you out of your hard earned cash!

There was a recent news story that frustrated me regarding the ingredients and contents of supplements that in all honesty, is truly despicable to the core. A football player years ago, having of performance enhancing drug use, had begun using a certain brand of protein shake, nothing harmful right, or so he thought. At the date of the routine drug test for the league, he received a notification saying he failed the test. In response, he was suspended from the team. This startled and frustrated him, he went and appealed to those that operated the test about how the results must have been mistaken. The analysts investigated all he would consume on a daily basis and analyzed his protein drink mix. Bingo! That was it! Apparently, at the factory of production of this particular supplement line, someone had mixed in an illegal substance into the protein batch. Furious, yet relieved and awakened by this revelation, this player expected to immediately be reinstated and to have his folly forgiven. This wasn't the case and he was forced to pay the price,   taking time out of his promising football career simply because of the actions of someone in a faraway factory or corporate office that advised to put this particular mixture in the protein product that was deemed "safe." The moral of the story is to be an informed and cautious individual when it comes to these such purchases.

Now, you might think that I'm completely "anti-supplement," which is highly inaccurate. I agree that supplements are necessary to aid in the muscle growth process, however, there are only a few brands that I've personally used and regard as reliable. Let me just say first that I only use BCAA's, glutamine, and typical whey protein, so I'm not as heavy user as others in this field. However, these brands are the ones that I have had personal experience and success with over the years, those being Cytosport, Myogenix, and Dymatize. I'm sure there are other great brands, but these are some of my favorites in regards to practicality and effectiveness. Cytosport whey protein is an affordable option, but just be key to track it as there is a moderate amount of sodium that comprises it, but for a cheaper option, it is definitely the way to go. What I currently use is Myogenix Whey Protein (https://www.amazon.com/gp/product/B0147Q84AK?ie=UTF8&tag=jchapman4z-20&camp=1789&linkCode=xm2&creativeASIN=B0147Q84AK) . This is known for its lower sugar and sodium content than other brands, which is why I prefer this to other, the downside is that is not as well known as Cytosport's Whey Protein product, but continually referring to these links should aid that process in finding the right supplements that builds your gains! (https://www.amazon.com/gp/product/B00DKRTCOK?ie=UTF8&tag=jchapman4z-20&camp=1789&linkCode=xm2&creativeASIN=B00DKRTCOK) . Lastly, the number one Glutamine distributor, in my opinion at least, is from Dymatize (https://www.amazon.com/gp/product/B0014NW9LK?ie=UTF8&tag=jchapman4z-20&camp=1789&linkCode=xm2&creativeASIN=B0014NW9LK) . Their product always has a large quantity of the supplement and is not going to break your piggy bank either.

In all, be the wise gladiator and use the guidance above to help navigate and protect you from the possibilities of manipulation that so many new trainees fall victim to. Use common sense and consult this chapter again if you have to in order to help you be a better informed user of these products! Don't let those people take advantage of your early on confusion and ambition!

Chapter 8

Suns Out, Guns Out?

Let's be honest guys, no matter whether you're out on the town, changing classes in school, or strolling around the office, if you want those gains to pop and be noticed, it's all in the clothes you decide to wear. There's a good bit of clothing hacks available to make yourself appear more muscular, hacks that everyone looking to have their physique stand out should know. Now just because this fashion illusion and tricks that we are creating may prove to help you a bit doesn't mean you should disregard the gym, these tricks are simply available to maximize the hard work that you have been putting in with your training and diet. I'll also cover the best places to find these affordable options and how to properly taper and style them if need be. Let's get rolling!

Number one, when ordering a short sleeve shirt or a t-shirt in general there are a few options that i have personally found great that make my body stand out as bigger and buffer. Those are the sleeve fit, the way it sticks to the chest, and the just the overall fit that comes with this style. In the case of short sleeves, the sleeve should be up high and tight to the upper arm, giving a mass exposure to the triceps and half of the bicep. This will make your arms appear larger than they already are as the tighter fit will make your arms more exposed, allowing everyone to see those gains you've been training for pop out. Along with that, make sure the shirt doesn't come baggy at the chest, this will make your chest look tiny, and we really don't want anyone to think that! Make sure the shirt is either very tapered to your chest, or simply wear a tank top or v neck layer beneath your shirt that you are wearing. This will give you a "V-Taper" look. Henley's also provide a great opportunity for this appearance as they are actually designed to broaden one's chest. Last, but not least, the size of the shirt is important. It may sound simple, but here it is, if you are a small shirt body type, don't buy a medium or a large! Simple as that! I see guys all the time who just waste their money on too large shirts that make them look tiny and scrawny. Please, for your own sake, by your own size, you'll be amazed at how everything falls into place when you do.

In regards to formal attire, always make sure that the clothing is in a slim fit style or athletic fit style! I personally only order slim fit sizes when I order my dress shirts or dress pants, shoot, even my polo shirts are slim fit. Having those items slim fit are the ticket. I'm serious, in all honesty, I can credit that particular style of fit for many of the outfit compliments that I have gotten out in public or from pictures of when I attended school dances. The fit of the outfit can make up for so many style blunders! Consider if you wore an ugly, and believe me I'm talking hideous purple dress shirt with a boring black tie, you could probably be regarded, or even get complimented if the style fit was proper. It's that simple, while coordination in an outfit is important, the fit is what makes it suitable for viewing. Always remember that when you consider a purchase of such clothes throughout your life, because formal style is inevitable, you'll always need it for some reason.

Now you are probably asking, "Well Jesse, I want to look good in my clothes and follow this guide, but I can't find anything and if I do, the price is way too expensive! What do I do?" Well lucky for you readers I'm the owner of a company specifically designed to solve that problem! Visit gentlemansdresser.com! I designed the site specifically for the modern day gladiators like us! Every outfit is slim fit and even the accessories are purposefully created to enhance your attractive features and make yourself show off that studly personality you've been working on! Go there, find something that really peaks your interest and treat yourself! Not only that, if you join the email list, we'll put you in the loop for special deals and discounts! There is absolutely no way to lose in this scenario. Yes, I'm self-advertising, but it's not about the sales to me, it's about how your life can go from zero to hero, just like mine did! If I had found a website like gentlemansdresser.com years ago, my road to becoming a modern day gladiator would have been so much easier! So to save you readers the strife, I made my own company for people like us! Pick up your attire today!

Chapter 9

Be Proud of Your Hard Work

Far too often I see people always seem to look down on others that have something better going for them. Whether it be a financial success, a healthy relationship, or as in our case gladiators, a better body than others. Rather than just accept defeat and let those that look down on people like us achieve a moral victory, we must honestly own the fact that we have a nice body. Why work so hard and not show the world? It makes plenty of sense to me in all honesty. If a person labors hard on crafting, they always show and display their results, if someone works hard on their car for days, they show off the results, why shouldn't we? If anything our commitments to our diets and regimes require more willpower, motivation, and consistency than any other of these well respected hobbies, so why should we be less proud. I'm not saying that we should be a bunch of arrogant douchebags, but if we want to post a shirtless selfie or walk around the beach and show the world our aesthetics, shouldn't we be allowed to do so without negative scrutiny? This journey is a long and treacherous one, we should be confident of ourselves and not hide our hard work!

Personally, I've had to deal with many negative people that would just mock and berate my physique. I'd see them in the gym, doing their ego lifting, fake macho style of training, acting like tough guys and being extremely rude to me because I don't train like them. Even on Snapchat and Instagram, to this day, I still get hate from people who share my photos around with negative intent. For the longest time, I let these people get a hold on my life and significantly affect my thinking, however, I later came to a realization. That realization was key and can be applied to anything. It simply was that these people are ignorant of the training process, sacrifice, and work ethic. These people were the kind to scoff when they see someone better off than they are. They are negative people who simply try to place themselves above others by tearing people down. This case isn't specific to me, there are individuals like this around the world. The question is, how do you make these people quit? It's simple, don't give them any power in your life. Seriously! That's all it takes. You have the power to control you and every single action you have, don't be reactive, take the proactive approach and don't let those kinds of people ruin your passion, they don't have the aspirations that you have for yourself, set don't let them dictate the way you live your life.

Now being proud and showing off those gains is awesome, but there's a difference between having fun with fitness and being a total douchebag. It's simple, respect other people while you're in your fun mode or zone, but don't rub it in anyone's face, that's how you make enemies out of people. Act in a way that will inspire people and not tear them down, once they see that, they will realize and respect what you do and the sacrifices that you have made to make your dream possible. The perspectives of the masses are simply controlled by the way we sell ourselves as characters and individuals. Sell and brand yourself the best possible way and you will gain such a great following from people that nobody will be able to bash or mock you in any way. Always value your character first and let that value show through your actions and enjoyment of your new found body.

In conclusion, these methods will play significantly into bolstering what is attracted around you. By cutting out and disregarding the negative people that have nothing positive to say, your potential growth is already appreciating, likewise, allowing people to see the beautiful creature and individual you have become allows for even better heights for you to reach! It makes sense on paper and sounds so simple, so why doesn't everyone apply that? It's sad, but easy to explain, most individuals simply don't encompass that kind of will power. They really struggle to let go of what some people, who literally have no bearing on their lives whatsoever, say about them. We all have had issues with this, but the power of proactive reaction allows us to already predetermine that we will block out these people. Utilize this skill, not just in a fitness sense, but in every life area as well, then, you will notice and feel the changes as you progress throughout your daily routines and habits. Don't let people who aren't gladiators hold you back!

Chapter 10

You're A Gladiator!!

So what should you take away from this book? You should understand that most things that people imply about fitness and its benefits being too difficult to achieve is complete horse manure. People are simply just looking for that instant gratification and so called "quick-fix" to help push them over the edge. As we've discussed, such a thing does not exist. Adapting a go-getter mentality will not only help you on the fitness end of your goal, it will boost you and build character for the rest of your life.

Many people just view fitness as a young man's game, but if you're older there is no need to quit. Likewise, there shouldn't be a reason that you shouldn't be able to start early either. You make it what you can and you will do what you aspire to. Forget the haters that mock and talk trash, you have goals and they don't. They aren't gladiators, they're jeering peasants, never take people like them seriously.

Unleash your inner beast in the gym! Do all you can do with maximum effort! Push yourself harder than anyone to get results and the results will come! I just want to leave you with one final thing, and yes, this is a short ending chapter, but here it is. Why would you ever want to quit when you look as good as you do? Stick with it and live life to the fullest. Show those girls that rejected you what they're missing out on! Show those gym punks who looks better! It's your time to rise! Let's go you gladiator!

Jeremiah 29:11